I0436505

OPTIMIZING DIGESTIVE HEALTH

Advanced Therapies For Gastrointestinal Wellness

Delve Into Effective Strategies For Maintaining A Healthy Digestive System, From Common Issues To Chronic Conditions

DR. BRIDGET PROMISE

Table of Contents

CHAPTER ONE 4

    Introduction 4

    Understanding The Digestive........................5

    Common Digestive Issues 7

CHAPTER TWO 10

    The Importance Of Diet In 10

    Nutritional Strategies For Digestive 12

CHAPTER THREE 19

    Probiotics And Gut Microbiota: 19

    Digestive Enzymes And Their 21

    Herbal Treatments For Digestive 23

    Stress Management For A Healthy 26

CHAPTER FOUR 30

    Physical Activity And Its Effect On 30

    Hydration For Improved Digestive...............33

    Food Allergies And Sensitivities 35

    Diagnostic Tools For.....................................37

CHAPTER FIVE 41

    Medical Treatments For Digestive 41

    Lifestyle Changes For 44

Holistic Approaches To Digestive.................45

Maintaining Digestive Health.......................49

Conclusion...52

CHAPTER ONE

Introduction

The digestive system is a vast and complicated network inside our bodies that converts food into nutrients that power our everyday activities and promote general health.

Understanding the digestive tract, frequent difficulties that may emerge, and the importance of nutrition in digestive health is critical for maintaining maximum well-being. In this investigation, we will dive into the complexities of the digestive system, throw light on common digestive disorders, and explain how dietary choices play an important part in supporting gastrointestinal health.

Understanding The Digestive System

The digestive system is a wonder of physiological engineering, consisting of a network of organs and systems that work together to process the food we eat. The process starts in the mouth, where mastication and saliva start the breakdown of carbs. The chewed meal goes down the esophagus to the stomach, where gastric acids further digest the contents. The partly digested meal reaches the small intestine, where the bulk of nutrients are absorbed. The remaining indigestible material enters the large intestine, where it absorbs water and forms the final waste product before being eliminated.

Several important organs contribute to the digestive process, with each having a unique function. The liver generates bile, which aids in fat digestion, while the pancreas secretes digestive enzymes that assist in breaking down proteins, fats, and carbs. The gallbladder stores and excretes bile as required. The enteric nervous system, often known as the "second brain," coordinates the whole process and controls digestive functions independent of the central nervous system.

Common Digestive Issues

Despite the precise architecture of the digestive system, a variety of variables may contribute to common digestive problems that impact millions of people worldwide. Indigestion, bloating, gas, constipation, diarrhea, and more serious disorders like irritable bowel syndrome (IBS) or inflammatory bowel disease (IBD) are all symptoms of gastrointestinal difficulties.

Understanding these difficulties is critical for detecting symptoms and getting the necessary treatment.

Overeating, eating spicy or fatty meals, or being stressed may all cause indigestion, which is characterized by pain and a burning feeling in the upper belly. Bloating and gas are induced by the fermentation of undigested food in the colon, which produces gasses. Constipation and diarrhea may indicate abnormal bowel habits or underlying gastrointestinal problems.

Chronic diseases such as IBS and IBD have long-term effects on gut health. IBS, a functional gastrointestinal illness, is characterized by stomach discomfort, bloating, and irregular bowel movements. IBD, on the other hand, includes disorders like Crohn's disease and ulcerative colitis, which cause inflammation in the digestive system and may lead to serious consequences.

CHAPTER TWO
The Importance Of Diet In Digestive Health

Diet has a significant impact on digestive health and function. Our dietary choices may either help or impede the complex processes involved in nutrient breakdown and absorption. A balanced and nutritious diet helps to maintain a healthy gut, but poor dietary choices may cause digestive pain and long-term health problems.

High-fiber meals, such as fruits, vegetables, and whole grains, stimulate regular bowel movements and help to maintain a healthy microbiome—the varied collection of bacteria that live in the gut. Probiotics, which are found in fermented foods such as yogurt, kefir, and sauerkraut, bring helpful bacteria into the digestive system, promoting digestion and immunological function.

Adequate hydration is necessary for digestion because water aids in the breakdown of food and its passage through the digestive system. Insufficient water consumption may cause constipation and impair the body's capacity to absorb nutrients efficiently.

In contrast, a diet heavy in processed foods, poor in fiber, and high in saturated fats might lead to digestive problems. Excessive intake of spicy or acidic meals may worsen problems such as acid reflux. Furthermore, artificial chemicals and preservatives in processed meals may disturb the gut microbiota, possibly causing inflammation and discomfort.

Nutritional Strategies For Digestive Wellness

Specific dietary practices are essential for promoting and maintaining gastrointestinal well-being. Here are some important factors for promoting digestive health with food choices:

1. Fiber-Rich Foods: Eat a range of fiber-rich foods, including whole grains, legumes, fruits and vegetables. Fiber encourages regular bowel movements, avoids constipation, and fosters the development of healthy bacteria in the stomach.

2. Consume probiotic-rich foods such as yogurt, kefir, kimchi, and kombucha in your diet. Probiotics contribute to a healthy balance of gut flora, promoting appropriate digestion and immunological function.

3. Hydration: Stay hydrated by drinking lots of water throughout the day. Water helps with digestion and vitamin absorption, which improves overall gastrointestinal health.

4. Limit your consumption of processed foods heavy in chemicals, preservatives, and harmful fats. These may alter the gut microbiome's normal equilibrium and cause stomach problems.

5. Mindful Eating: Enjoy each mouthful, chew carefully, and pay attention to hunger and fullness signs. This improves regular

digestion and helps to avoid overeating.

6. Moderate Spicy and Acidic Meals: Limit your intake of spicy and acidic meals, particularly if you suffer from acid reflux or heartburn. These may irritate the esophagus, causing pain.

7. Identify Food Sensitivities: Pay attention to how your body reacts to various foods and look for possible sensitivities. Dairy, gluten, and specific FODMAPs (fermentable oligosaccharides, disaccharides, monosaccharides, and polyols) are all common causes.

8. Balanced Meals: Aim for meals that include a variety of carbs, proteins, and healthy fats. This ensures a consistent flow of nutrients and energy, promoting proper digestion.

9. Regular Physical Activity: Exercise supports good digestion and helps to avoid constipation. Even mild exercises, such as walking, may improve gastrointestinal function.

10. Practice stress-reduction strategies like meditation, deep breathing, or yoga. Chronic stress may influence digestive health,

resulting in illnesses such as irritable bowel syndrome.

In conclusion, the digestive system is critical to overall health, and knowing its complexities is essential for supporting gastrointestinal well-being. Common digestive difficulties may frequently be addressed by making thoughtful dietary choices that prioritize fiber-rich foods, probiotics, water, and a well-balanced diet. Individuals who follow these dietary guidelines may take proactive actions to ensure that their digestive systems work well, therefore boosting their general well-being.

The complex link between our digestive system and general well-being is a growing issue of interest and study in the field of holistic health. Understanding the interactions between probiotics, gut bacteria, digestive enzymes, herbal medicines, and stress management is critical for maintaining a healthy gut and, by extension, a flourishing body.

CHAPTER THREE

Probiotics And Gut Microbiota:

Probiotics, sometimes known as "good bacteria," are living microorganisms that provide health advantages when taken at suitable levels.

These beneficial bacteria typically live in the gastrointestinal system, constituting what is known as the gut microbiome. The gut microbiota is a complex and dynamic community of trillions of microorganisms, including bacteria, viruses, fungi, and other microbes.

Probiotics are essential for maintaining the delicate equilibrium of this microbial ecosystem. They improve the general health of the digestive tract by encouraging the development of healthy bacteria and reducing harmful microbes. Probiotics are present in a variety of fermented foods, including yogurt, kefir, sauerkraut, and kimchi, as well as supplements.

According to research, a well-balanced and diversified gut microbiota is necessary for proper digestion, nutritional absorption, and immunity.

Dysbiosis, or imbalances in the gut microbiota, has been related to a variety of digestive problems, immunological illnesses, and even mental health difficulties. Incorporating probiotic-rich foods or supplements into one's diet might be a proactive step toward maintaining a healthy gut environment.

Digestive Enzymes And Their Importance

Digestive enzymes are proteins generated by the body that help break down food into smaller, more absorbable components. These enzymes are released at numerous locations throughout the digestive system, including the mouth, stomach, and small intestine. Each enzyme is designed to break down a certain nutrient, such as carbs, proteins, or lipids.

Amylase, for example, helps break down carbs into sugars, whereas protease digests proteins and lipase digests lipids. Insufficient digestive enzyme synthesis may cause nutritional malabsorption, resulting in bloating, gas, and other digestive discomforts.

Certain variables, such as age, stress, and medical problems, might impair the body's capacity to create enough digestive enzymes. In such circumstances, enzyme supplements may be beneficial in supporting the digestive process and alleviating indigestion symptoms. Enzyme-rich foods such as pineapple and papaya may also help with digestion naturally.

Herbal Treatments For Digestive Support:

Nature has offered a profusion of herbs that have long been utilized for digestive purposes. Ginger is well-known for its ability to calm the digestive system, ease nausea, and reduce inflammation.

Peppermint is another plant that has a relaxing impact on the digestive tract, which may help ease symptoms of indigestion and irritable bowel syndrome.

Chamomile, which has mild anti-inflammatory qualities, is often drank as a tea to relieve stomach distress and induce relaxation. Fennel, cumin, and coriander, all frequent ingredients in traditional spice blends, are recognized for their carminative effects, which aid in relieving gas and bloating.

Herbal medicines are used for more than just symptom alleviation; certain herbs improve intestinal health in general. For example, licorice root has been investigated for its ability to strengthen the stomach's mucous lining, providing a protective barrier against gastric acid and encouraging healing in instances of gastritis or ulcers.

When adding herbal medicines to one's regimen, it is important to be aware of individual sensitivities and possible interactions with drugs. Consulting with a healthcare expert or herbalist may help you personalize herbal remedies to your unique requirements and health concerns.

Stress Management For A Healthy Gut:

The delicate relationship between the gut and the brain is often referred to as the "gut-brain axis." Stress, whether acute or chronic, may have a substantial influence on this axis, affecting the health and function of the digestive system.

The enteric nervous system, also known as the "second brain," is a complex network of neurons found in the stomach that interacts with the central nervous system in both directions.

When stress causes the "fight or flight" reaction, blood flow is diverted away from the digestive organs, resulting in reduced digestive function. Furthermore, stress may upset the equilibrium of gut flora, possibly leading to gastrointestinal problems.

Incorporating stress management practices into everyday life is consequently essential for gut health. Deep breathing techniques, meditation, yoga, and regular physical activity have all been demonstrated to benefit the gut-brain axis, encouraging calm and healthy digestion.

Furthermore, mindfulness-based stress reduction strategies may be especially useful for treating illnesses like irritable bowel syndrome (IBS) and inflammatory bowel disease (IBD). These techniques not only treat the physiological components of stress, but they also promote a comprehensive approach to well-being.

Finally, a comprehensive approach to digestive health requires a thorough knowledge of the interactions between probiotics, gut bacteria, digestive enzymes, herbal treatments, and stress management. By integrating these ingredients into our everyday lives, we may cultivate a healthy and flourishing gut, creating the groundwork for general health and energy.

CHAPTER FOUR
Physical Activity And Its Effect On Digestion

Physical exercise is essential for sustaining overall health, and its benefits extend beyond cardiovascular fitness and physical strength. Regular exercise has been linked to a variety of health advantages, including improved digestion.

The link between exercise and digestion is complex, comprising several physiological processes that contribute to proper gastrointestinal function.

When we participate in physical activity, particularly moderate-intensity workouts like walking, running, or cycling, our digestive system reacts in a variety of ways. One immediate impact is increased blood flow to digestive organs including the stomach and intestines. This increased blood circulation helps provide more oxygen and nutrients to these organs, encouraging optimum performance.

Physical exercise also promotes the contraction of muscles, particularly those in the gastrointestinal system. These contractions, known as peristalsis, help food pass through the digestive system more efficiently. The regular contractions drive food from the esophagus to the stomach and intestines, supporting efficient digestion and nutritional absorption.

Regular exercise has also been demonstrated to help regulate bowel motions, lowering the risk of constipation. Physical exercise tones the abdominal muscles, improving their capacity to support and transport the contents of the digestive system. This may be especially advantageous for those who suffer from gastrointestinal difficulties including irritable bowel syndrome (IBS) or constipation.

Hydration For Improved Digestive Function

Proper hydration is vital for general health and has a significant influence on digestive function. Water is an essential component of the digestive process, helping to break down food, absorb nutrients, and eliminate waste. When the body is properly hydrated, these processes run smoothly and effectively.

Water aids in the digestion of food particles in the stomach, allowing digestive enzymes to function more effectively. It also improves nutrition absorption in the small intestine. Insufficient water consumption may cause constipation because the colon absorbs water from the feces, making it harder to pass. Chronic dehydration may lead to long-term digestive problems, stressing the significance of drinking enough fluids regularly.

In addition to ordinary water, herbal teas and other liquids, such as broths, may help with general hydration and digestive health. However, excessive use of caffeinated or sugary drinks may have the opposite effect, perhaps causing dehydration and impairing digestion.

Food Allergies And Sensitivities

Food intolerances and sensitivities may have a substantial influence on digestive health. While the terms are often used interchangeably, there are significant distinctions between them.

dietary intolerances are primarily caused by the digestive system's inability to effectively break down certain dietary components. Lactose intolerance, for example, develops when the body lacks the enzyme lactase, which is responsible for breaking down lactose, a sugar present in milk and dairy products. Undigested lactose may cause symptoms including bloating, gas, and diarrhea.

diet sensitivities, on the other hand, are the immune system's reaction to certain proteins in the diet. Gluten sensitivity is a frequent condition in which the immune system responds to gluten, a protein present in wheat, barley, and rye. This immune reaction may cause inflammation and other gastrointestinal symptoms, such as stomach discomfort and diarrhea.

Identifying and controlling dietary intolerances and sensitivities is critical to digestive health. Individuals who are suffering from recurrent digestive problems should visit a healthcare expert or a trained dietitian for an accurate diagnosis and advice on how to manage their food choices.

Diagnostic Tools For Gastrointestinal Health

As medical technology has advanced, so has the diagnosis of gastrointestinal problems. Various diagnostic methods are used to analyze and comprehend the complexities of digestive health, assisting healthcare practitioners in identifying the underlying causes of digestive problems and developing successful treatment regimens.

Endoscopic procedures, such as esophagogastroduodenoscopy (EGD) and colonoscopy, enable doctors to see the lining of the digestive system. These procedures may assist in uncovering irregularities, inflammation, and other structural concerns that may be causing digestive problems.

Imaging methods such as computed tomography (CT) scans and magnetic resonance imaging (MRI) give comprehensive pictures of the abdomen and pelvic areas, which assist in the detection of diseases affecting organs such as the liver, gallbladder, and pancreas.

Laboratory studies, such as blood testing and stool analysis, are essential for determining intestinal health. Blood testing may detect signs of inflammation or nutritional inadequacies, while stool analysis can provide information on gastrointestinal function, such as malabsorption or the presence of aberrant microbes.

Functional diagnostic techniques, such as hydrogen breath tests, may help diagnose disorders including small intestine bacterial overgrowth (SIBO) and specific carbohydrate malabsorption. These tests evaluate the gasses generated by bacteria in the digestive system, providing information on the balance of microorganisms and their effects on digestion.

CHAPTER FIVE

Medical Treatments For
Digestive Diseases

When lifestyle and nutritional changes are insufficient, medical intervention is required to manage and treat digestive issues. The choice of intervention is determined by the exact diagnosis and severity of the ailment.

To treat gastroesophageal reflux disease (GERD), drugs such as proton pump inhibitors (PPIs) may be used to lower stomach acid production and relieve symptoms. Other drugs used to treat acid-related digestive disorders include antacids and H2 blockers.

Inflammatory bowel illnesses (IBD), such as Crohn's disease and ulcerative colitis, may need a mix of treatments, including anti-inflammatory agents, immunosuppressives, and biologics. These drugs try to reduce inflammation and manage symptoms, enabling people with IBD to live more comfortably.

Certain digestive diseases that may not respond well to medicine or lifestyle modifications may warrant surgical intervention. In certain circumstances, laparoscopic gallbladder removal (cholecystectomy) or colon surgery to treat problems such as diverticulitis may be suggested.

To summarize, sustaining gut health requires a comprehensive strategy that includes physical exercise, water, knowledge of dietary intolerances and sensitivities, proper diagnostic tools, and medicinal therapies as needed. Understanding the complicated relationships between lifestyle, nutrition, and digestive function allows people to manage their digestive health proactively and treat difficulties as they arise, resulting in greater overall well-being.

Lifestyle Changes For Gastrointestinal Wellness

Digestive health is an important component of total well-being, affecting not just our physical health but also our mental and emotional moods. Incorporating lifestyle changes that promote gut well-being may have long-term advantages. Holistic methods highlight the interconnectivity of numerous digestion-related aspects, resulting in a holistic framework for digestive health.

Holistic Approaches To Digestive Health

Holistic health acknowledges the delicate link between the mind, body, and spirit, stressing the significance of treating the full person rather than just the symptoms. When it comes to gastrointestinal health, holistic methods go beyond nutrition and exercise, recognizing the influence of stress, sleep, and emotional well-being on digestive function.

1. Mindful Eating: Mindful eating is essential for maintaining overall digestive health. This is being completely present throughout

meals, appreciating each mouthful, and responding to hunger and fullness signs. Individuals who eat slowly and enjoy the sensory experience of food may improve digestion and nutrient absorption.

2. Stress Management: Chronic stress may negatively impact digestive health, causing symptoms including indigestion, bloating, and IBS. Stress management practices, such as meditation, deep breathing exercises, and yoga, may benefit the digestive tract. These techniques encourage relaxation,

lowering the risk of stress-related gastrointestinal disorders.

3. Proper Hydration: Staying hydrated is crucial for good digestive function. Water aids in the digestion of food, the absorption of nutrients, and the smooth passage of waste through the digestive system. Drinking enough water throughout the day will help you avoid constipation and improve your overall gut health.

4. Regular physical activity promotes digestive health. Physical exercise stimulates the muscles of the digestive system,

encouraging regular bowel movements and reducing constipation. Furthermore, exercise helps with weight control, lowering the risk of obesity-related digestive problems such as acid reflux and gallstones.

5. Incorporating probiotics and prebiotics into your diet may improve gut health. Probiotics are good bacteria that help to balance the gut microbiota, while prebiotics are non-digestible carbohydrates that feed these beneficial bacteria. Yogurt, kefir, sauerkraut, and fiber-rich fruits and vegetables may help maintain a healthy gut flora.

Maintaining Digestive Health Long-Term

Sustainable adjustments are critical for long-term gut health. Adopting a proactive approach and incorporating these changes into everyday life may have a substantial impact on overall well-being.

1. A balanced and diverse diet is essential for digestive health. Include a wide variety of fruits, vegetables, whole grains, lean meats, and healthy fats in your meals. Fiber-rich diets, in particular, encourage regular

bowel motions and support a healthy gut environment.

2. Identifying and restricting trigger foods might help individuals with digestive sensitivities or illnesses like IBS or acid reflux. Caffeine, alcohol, spicy foods, and high-fat meals are all common causes. Keeping a food journal may help you detect trends and make educated dietary decisions.

3. Regular Check-Ups: Regular medical check-ups are vital for detecting and treating any potential stomach problems. Regular screenings may spot

abnormalities early on, allowing for prompt action and the avoidance of more serious illnesses. Consult a healthcare practitioner if you have any chronic digestive issues or concerns.

4. Moderate Eating Habits: Overeating may strain the digestive system, causing pain and even long-term problems. Portion management, avoiding late-night meals, and allowing the digestive system enough time to absorb food before sleep are all important behaviors for maintaining good digestive health.

5. Quality Sleep: Getting enough sleep improves general health, including digestion. Establishing a regular sleep schedule and getting enough sleep might improve gastrointestinal health.

Conclusion

Incorporating lifestyle changes for gastrointestinal wellness is a comprehensive strategy that tackles the many aspects that influence digestive health. Mindful diet, stress management, hydration, regular physical exercise, and the use of probiotics and prebiotics all contribute to an overall digestive health plan. Furthermore, long-term maintenance of these changes, coupled with a balanced diet, minimizing trigger foods, frequent check-ups, moderation in eating behaviors, and emphasizing excellent sleep, promotes long-term health advantages.

Individuals may empower themselves by understanding the complex link between lifestyle choices and digestive health, allowing them to make proactive efforts toward achieving a harmonic balance in their bodies. The quest for good gut health is continuous, and adopting a holistic approach may lead to a happier, more vibrant existence.

www.ingramcontent.com/pod-product-compliance
Lightning Source LLC
Chambersburg PA
CBHW070848310526
45796CB00014B/256